Healthy Gut, Healthy Life

A Simplified Guide with Simple Strategies to Improve Your Well-Being with Probiotics, Fiber-Rich Foods, and Easy Lifestyle Changes

Daisy Houle

Table Of Contents

Foreword
Introduction to the Gut Microbiome

Let's start at the beginning· The gut microbiome is like a big community of tiny organisms living in our digestive system· These tiny organisms include bacteria, viruses, fungi, and tiny creatures called protozoa· They're not just hanging out; they do a lot of work for us· They help us digest our food, make vitamins we need, protect us from bad germs, and can even affect how we feel and think·

From the time we're born, these tiny organisms start to make a home in our gut· What we eat, how we live, and the places we're in can change this tiny world inside us· It's like a garden that grows differently based on how we take care of it·

Having the right balance of these tiny organisms is key to keeping us healthy· If the balance is off, we might not feel well· This book will teach you the basics about these tiny organisms and why they're so important for our health·

We'll make everything easy to understand, so you can learn how taking care of your gut can help you feel better and healthier· Let's get started on this journey to better health by learning how to take care of the tiny organisms that do so much for us·

Part I: Understanding the Gut Microbiome

What Is the Gut Microbiome?

The gut microbiome refers to the vast community of microorganisms living in our digestive system. Imagine it as a bustling city within our bodies, where trillions of bacteria, viruses, fungi, and protozoa thrive together. This community is not just a passive presence; it plays an active role in our health. These microorganisms help break down food, make vitamins, fight off harmful germs, and even influence our mood and weight. Each person's gut microbiome is unique, like a fingerprint, but all are essential for maintaining good health.

Historical Perspective and Recent Discoveries

The study of the gut microbiome is not new, but our understanding has grown exponentially in recent years· Initially, scientists knew that our bodies hosted microbes, but they didn't understand the extent of their influence on our health and well-being· Early research focused on harmful bacteria until the advent of modern technology allowed us to see the beneficial aspects of our microbial inhabitants·

In the past, scientists could only study microbes that could be grown in labs, which was a small fraction of the gut's microbial population· However, with the development of DNA sequencing technologies, we've been able to explore the gut microbiome more fully· These advances have unveiled the microbiome's critical role in digestion, immunity, and even mental health, leading to a surge in research aimed at understanding how these microbes influence our health and how we can support them in return·

Recent discoveries have highlighted the gut microbiome's link to diseases such as obesity, type 2 diabetes, irritable bowel syndrome, and even depression· This has shifted the view of the microbiome from a simple ecosystem to a complex, influential factor in our overall health· Researchers have also begun to explore how diet, antibiotics, and lifestyle changes can impact the microbiome for better or worse, opening the door to new approaches in health care and disease prevention·

This part of the book lays the groundwork for understanding the intricate relationship between our bodies and the microorganisms that reside within us· It sets the stage for a deeper dive into how we can nurture this relationship for optimal health, underscoring the microbiome's significance not just as a fascinating scientific frontier but as a pivotal component of our daily health and well-being·

The Science of the Gut

Understanding how the gut works are crucial for grasping the broader implications of gut health on overall well-being· The gut, often referred to as the gastrointestinal (GI) tract, is a complex system responsible for digesting food, absorbing nutrients, and expelling waste· It begins at the mouth and extends through the esophagus, stomach, small intestine, and large intestine, ending at the rectum and anus· Each segment plays a specific role in digestion, from the initial breakdown of food with saliva in the mouth to the absorption of nutrients in the small intestine and the formation and excretion of waste in the large intestine·

How the Gut Works

When we eat, our gut springs into action· Food is broken down mechanically by chewing and chemically by digestive enzymes· In the stomach, this mixture becomes a semi-liquid substance called chyme, which then moves to the small intestine· Here, the majority of nutrient absorption occurs through tiny, finger-like projections called villi· The gut microbiome interacts with this process by breaking down fibers and other components that our human cells can't digest, producing vitamins and other essential nutrients in the process·

The gut also has a protective role· The intestinal lining acts as a barrier, preventing harmful substances and pathogens from entering the bloodstream· The microbiome supports this function by competing with harmful bacteria for resources and stimulating the immune system·

The Gut-Brain Axis: A Two-Way Communication

One of the most fascinating aspects of gut science is the gut-brain axis, a complex communication network linking the gut and the brain· This relationship allows the gut and brain to send signals to each other, influencing not just digestive functions but also emotional and cognitive states·

The gut-brain axis operates through various pathways, including the nervous system, hormones, and the immune system· For instance, the vagus nerve, one of the largest nerves connecting the gut and the brain, transmits signals in both directions· This explains why stress can upset your stomach or why gut disorders can be linked to anxiety and depression·

Recent research has shown that the gut microbiome plays a significant role in this communication· Certain microbes can produce neurotransmitters, such as serotonin and dopamine, which are crucial for mood regulation· These substances can signal the brain and influence our emotions, stress levels, and even pain perception·

Understanding the gut-brain axis opens up new perspectives on the impact of gut health beyond digestion· It highlights the importance of a healthy gut microbiome for mental health and provides a scientific basis for the concept of "gut feelings·" This knowledge paves the way for novel treatments for both gut disorders and mental health conditions, emphasizing the need for a holistic approach to health that considers the intricate connections between our gut and brain.

The Role of Microbiome in Health and Disease

Our gut is filled with tiny living things, like bacteria and fungi, that help us stay healthy· These tiny creatures form what we call the microbiome· They do a lot for us, from helping us digest food to fighting off sickness· But when they're out of balance, it can lead to health problems·

Immunity and the Microbiome

The microbiome helps our body's defence system, or immune system, know what to fight off and what to leave alone· It's like teaching a puppy what is a toy and what is not· This helps us not get sick from germs and stops our body from attacking itself, which can happen in some diseases· The good bacteria in our gut also make a wall that stops bad germs from getting into our blood·

The Microbiome and Chronic Diseases

When the balance of good and bad bacteria in our gut is off, it can lead to long-lasting health problems, like being overweight, having diabetes, heart disease, and stomach problems· For example, if we have too many of a certain type of bacteria, it might make our body hold onto fat more or mess with our sugar levels· It can also cause inflammation, which is our body's way of fighting off what it thinks are invaders but can make us sick if there's too much·

Mental Health and the Gut-Brain Connection

Our gut and brain talk to each other through a special connection. This means that how our gut feels can affect our mood. Scientists have found that people who are very sad or worried sometimes have different bacteria in their gut than people who aren't. The bacteria in our gut can make chemicals that affect our brain, like serotonin, which makes us feel happy. So, keeping our gut bacteria happy can help us feel happier, too.

In simple terms, the tiny creatures in our gut are super important for our health, not just for our stomach but for our whole body and mind. Eating healthy foods, like fruits, vegetables, and foods with good bacteria (like yoghurt), can help keep our gut and us healthy.

Part II: Factors Affecting the Gut Microbiome

Diet and the Microbiome

The connection between what we eat and the health of our gut microbiome is profound and complex. Every bite of food we take is not just nourishment for us, but also for the trillions of microorganisms residing in our digestive tract. These microorganisms are essential players in our health, influencing everything from digestion and nutrient absorption to immune function and even our mood.

How Diet Influences Gut Health

Our diet acts as the primary source of energy and nutrients for our gut microbiome. You can think of your gut as a bustling city where the inhabitants—various bacteria, fungi, and other microorganisms—have diverse dietary preferences· Just as a city thrives when its residents have access to a wide variety of resources, our gut microbiome flourishes on a diverse and nutrient-rich diet·

Eating a diet rich in fruits, vegetables, legumes, and whole grains provides a broad spectrum of fibers, vitamins, and minerals that support a diverse microbial population· This diversity is key to a resilient gut ecosystem, capable of withstanding challenges like infections and helping to break down foodstuffs that our bodies can't digest on their own·

Conversely, a diet high in processed foods, sugars, and unhealthy fats can disrupt this delicate balance· Such foods can promote the growth of harmful bacteria and yeasts, leading to a decrease in microbial diversity and an increase in gut inflammation· Over time, this imbalance can contribute to a range of health issues, including digestive disorders, obesity, and even mental health conditions·

Probiotics and Prebiotics: What's the Difference?

To further support our gut microbiome, we can turn to probiotics and prebiotics, both of which play unique roles in maintaining gut health·

Probiotics are live beneficial bacteria that add to the population of good microbes in our gut· They're like new, friendly residents moving into the gut city, helping to maintain a healthy community· Fermented food such as yoghurt, kefir, sauerkraut, and kimchi are rich in these beneficial bacteria· Regularly incorporating these foods into our diet can help replenish and diversify the good bacteria in our gut, aiding in

digestion, nutrient absorption, and immune
function.

Prebiotics, on the other hand, are the food that
our gut bacteria eat. They are a type of non-
digestible fiber found in foods like bananas,
onions, garlic, asparagus, and whole grains.
Eating a diet rich in prebiotics can help fuel the
good bacteria in our gut, allowing them to
multiply and thrive. This is akin to planting
more trees and plants in a city to provide more
oxygen and improve the quality of life for its
residents.

In essence, maintaining a healthy gut
microbiome through diet involves both
introducing beneficial bacteria via probiotics
and feeding those bacteria with prebiotics. This
synergistic approach supports a vibrant, diverse

microbial community in our gut, which in turn supports our overall health·

By understanding and applying these principles, we can make dietary choices that promote a healthy gut microbiome· This, in turn, can have far-reaching effects on our health, from enhancing our digestive system and immune response to potentially improving our mood and cognitive function· The food we eat directly influences the complex ecosystem within us, emphasizing the adage "you are what you eat" in a very literal sense·

Lifestyle and Environmental Impacts

Our gut health is not only influenced by what we eat but also by our lifestyle choices and the environment around us· From the amount of stress we experience to how much we move and sleep, every aspect of our daily lives can have a profound impact on the microbiome within us· Additionally, the medications we take, especially antibiotics, can have lasting effects on our gut health·

Stress and Sleep: Their Effect on the Gut

Stress is a normal part of life, but chronic stress can wreak havoc on our gut microbiome· When we're stressed, our body releases hormones that can alter the gut environment, making it less friendly for good bacteria· This shift can lead to a decrease in microbial diversity and an increase in harmful bacteria· Chronic stress may also increase gut permeability, often referred to as "leaky gut," allowing bacteria and toxins to enter the bloodstream, which can lead to inflammation and other health issues·

Sleep plays a critical role in maintaining a healthy gut· Just as our body needs rest to function properly, our gut microbes also follow a daily rhythm· Disruptions in our sleep patterns, like staying up late or shift work, can disturb the natural cycle of our gut bacteria, leading to imbalances· Adequate, restful sleep supports the diversity and health of the gut microbiome, which in turn can influence our sleep quality, creating a beneficial cycle·

Exercise and the Microbiome

Exercise has a positive impact on the gut microbiome· Regular physical activity can increase the diversity of our gut bacteria, which is a key indicator of good gut health· Exercise promotes the growth of beneficial bacteria that can improve the integrity of the gut barrier, reduce inflammation, and enhance overall immune function· Whether it's a daily walk, a run, or a yoga session, incorporating regular physical activity into our routine can significantly benefit our gut health and, by extension, our overall well-being·

Antibiotics and Medications: A Double-Edged Sword

Antibiotics are essential for fighting bacterial infections, but they can also have unintended consequences on our gut microbiome· While they target harmful bacteria, antibiotics can also kill off beneficial bacteria, disrupting the delicate balance within our gut· This disruption can lead to a decrease in microbial diversity and make room for harmful bacteria to grow, potentially leading to antibiotic-associated diarrhea or more serious conditions like Clostridium difficile infection·

Other medications, including non-steroidal anti-inflammatory drugs (NSAIDs), birth control pills, and acid reducers, can also impact the gut microbiome· These medications may alter the gut environment, affect bacterial growth, or change the composition of the microbiome, leading to imbalances·

The key is to use medications judiciously and under the guidance of a healthcare professional· After a course of antibiotics or other medications that may affect the gut, taking steps to restore the gut microbiome, such as consuming probiotics and prebiotics, can be beneficial.

In summary, our lifestyle choices and the environment play crucial roles in shaping our gut health. Managing stress, ensuring adequate sleep, engaging in regular exercise, and being mindful of medication use can all help support a healthy, balanced gut microbiome. By making conscious choices in these areas, we can foster a gut environment that supports our overall health and well-being.

Part III: Nourishing Your Gut Microbiome

The Foundation of a Gut-Healthy Diet

A diet that's good for your gut microbiome is like giving the best possible fuel to a car· It helps everything run smoothly· The right foods can help your gut bacteria thrive, which in turn keeps you healthy· Let's look at some basic rules for a diet that's friendly to the gut microbiome and discuss which foods to eat more of and which ones to limit·

Core Principles of a Microbiome-Friendly Diet

1. ***Diversity is Key:*** Just like a garden with many different types of plants is healthier, a varied diet helps to support a diverse microbiome· Eating a wide range

of foods, especially fruits, vegetables, legumes, and whole grains, can provide different types of fibers and nutrients that feed different beneficial bacteria in your gut.

2. ***Fiber is Your Friend:*** Fiber from plants is something our body can't digest, but our gut bacteria love it. Eating plenty of fiber-rich foods helps to feed the good bacteria, which break it down into important nutrients that our body can use. This process can also produce short-chain fatty acids that are great for our health.

3. ***Include Fermented Foods:*** Fermented foods are like a live supplement of good bacteria. Foods like yoghurt, kefir, sauerkraut, and kimchi add

beneficial bacteria to your gut, helping to increase its diversity and resilience·

4. ***Limit Sugar and Processed Foods:*** Foods high in sugar and processed foods can feed harmful bacteria and yeast, leading to an imbalance in your gut· Reducing these foods can help maintain a healthier microbiome·

5. ***Stay Hydrated:*** Drinking plenty of water has numerous health benefits, including keeping the lining of your gut healthy and supporting the growth of good bacteria·

Foods to Embrace and Avoid

Foods to Embrace:

<u>*Vegetables*</u>: All kinds, especially leafy greens and those rich in fiber like:

Leafy greens (spinach, kale)

Cruciferous vegetables (broccoli, cauliflower)

Root vegetables (carrots, beets)

More varieties like scallions, chives, sweet potatoes, squash, and pumpkin. Seaweeds like: Nori, kelp, and wakame, which offer unique marine-based fibers and nutrients·

<u>*Fruits:*</u> A variety of fruits provide vitamins, minerals, and fibers that beneficial bacteria need· Go for

A mix of berries, citrus fruits, apples, pears, and tropical fruits like mango and pineapple· other fruits you can include are peaches, plums, nectarines, watermelon, cantaloupe, honeydew, and pomegranates

<u>*Whole Grains:*</u> Foods like

Oats

Quinoa

Barley

Whole wheat, and brown rice provide complex carbohydrates that are great for your gut bacteria·

Ancient Grains: *Amaranth, spelt, and teff* offer additional fibre and nutrients·

Sprouted Grains and Nuts: Sprouting can increase nutrient availability and digestibility·

<u>Legumes:</u>

Beans (black beans, kidney beans)

Lentils, and chickpeas are a great sources of protein (plant-based) and fiber ·

<u>Nuts and Seeds:</u>

Almonds

Walnuts

Chia seeds

Flaxseeds, and pumpkin seeds.

These are good sources of fiber, healthy fats, and other nutrients that support gut health.

Fermented Foods: Incorporate foods like

Yoghurt

Kefir

Sauerkraut

Kombucha, and kimchi

to add beneficial bacteria to your diet.

Healthy Fats:

Avocados

Olive oil

Fatty fish (like mackerel and salmon)

offer omega-3 fatty acids that support gut health.

Herbs and Spices:

Turmeric

Ginger

Garlic, and cinnamon

can have anti-inflammatory effects on the gut.

Prebiotic Foods:
Asparagus
Bananas
Garlic
Onions, and leeks
feed the good bacteria in your gut.

Hydration:
Water
Herbal teas, and bone broth
support overall digestion and gut health.

Foods to Avoid or Limit:
High-Sugar Foods: Sugary snacks and beverages can promote the growth of harmful bacteria and yeasts. Foods like *Candy* *Sugary drinks, and pastries*

can lead to an overgrowth of harmful bacteria and yeast.

Processed and Refined Foods:
White bread
Pasta, and snacks
that lack dietary fiber and nutrients, often high in sugar, unhealthy fats, and additives that can disrupt the gut microbiome.

Artificial Sweeteners: Some studies suggest that artificial sweeteners can negatively affect the gut microbiome.

Red and Processed Meats: Consuming large amounts of these can be detrimental to gut health due to certain compounds that they contain.

Fried and High-Fat Foods: Foods high in unhealthy fats can contribute to inflammation and discomfort in the gut.

Alcohol: In moderation, some alcohols like red wine can be beneficial, but excessive consumption is harmful to gut health·

Dairy Products: Some individuals may need to limit dairy due to lactose intolerance or sensitivity affecting their gut·

Gluten-Containing Foods: Those with celiac disease or gluten sensitivity should avoid wheat, barley, and rye·

Caffeinated Beverages: Excessive caffeine can irritate the gut, especially for those with sensitive stomachs·

Artificial Additives: Preservatives, colourings, and flavourings in some processed foods can disrupt the gut microbiome·

Balancing your diet with foods to embrace while minimizing those to avoid can support a healthy, diverse gut microbiome· This not only aids in digestion and nutrient absorption but also plays a significant role in your overall health and well-being. Remember, individual tolerance varies, so it's essential to listen to your body and adjust your diet accordingly.

A gut-healthy diet is about making choices that support the diverse ecosystem within your gut. By focusing on nutrient-rich, fiber-dense, and fermented foods, you can help nourish your microbiome, which in turn supports your overall health. Remember, the goal is to create a diet that you enjoy and can stick with, which also promotes a healthy and diverse gut microbiome.

Incorporating Probiotics and Prebiotics

Fermented Foods and Beyond

Probiotics are the good bacteria that live in our gut and help us stay healthy. Think of them as friendly helpers that keep our digestive system running smoothly. We can add more of these helpful bacteria to our gut by eating fermented foods. Fermentation is a natural process where microorganisms like bacteria and yeast turn the sugars in food into acids or alcohol. This not only preserves the food but also creates these beneficial bacteria.

Some great examples of fermented foods include:

<u>**Yoghurt and Kefir:**</u> These dairy products are fermented with bacteria that are good for our

gut· Look for ones that say "live and active cultures" on the label·

Sauerkraut and Kimchi: Made from fermented cabbage and other vegetables, these foods are not only rich in probiotics but also vitamins and fiber ·

Pickles: When made through fermentation (not just in vinegar), pickles can be a source of good bacteria· Check how they're made to be sure·

Miso and Tempeh: These are fermented soy products popular in Asian cuisine, packed with probiotics and plant-based protein·
Eating a variety of these foods can help increase the number and variety of good bacteria in your gut·

The Power of Fiber: Vegetables, Fruits, and Whole Grains

Prebiotics are like the food for our friendly gut bacteria. They're a type of fiber that we, humans, can't digest, but our gut bacteria love to eat. By consuming prebiotic-rich foods, we can help nourish our gut bacteria, allowing them to thrive, multiply, and keep our gut healthy.

Foods rich in prebiotics include:

Vegetables: Especially those with lots of fiber like artichokes, garlic, onions, leeks, asparagus, and shallots. These veggies are not only nutritious but also packed with the kind of fiber that feeds our good bacteria.

Fruits: Bananas, apples (with the skin on), and berries are good choices. They offer a sweet treat plus a dose of fiber that supports gut health.

<u>Whole Grains:</u> Foods like oats, barley, and bran are full of fiber · Including these in your meals can help ensure your gut bacteria have plenty to eat·

By focusing on these fiber-rich foods, you're not just feeding yourself; you're also feeding the beneficial bacteria that live in your gut· This helps maintain a balanced and healthy digestive system, which is crucial for overall health·

Combining probiotics and prebiotics in your diet is like creating a perfect environment for a healthy gut· The probiotics add more good bacteria, and the prebiotics feed them, helping them to grow and flourish· This synergy supports not just a healthy digestive system but also strengthens your immune system and can improve your mood and energy levels· So, embracing a diet rich in both probiotics and prebiotics can lead to significant benefits for your health and well-being·

Hydration and Gut Health

Maintaining proper hydration is like ensuring the rivers and streams in a vast ecosystem flow smoothly, providing life and nourishment to the entire landscape. In the context of our body, water and other fluids play a crucial role in keeping our digestive system healthy and functioning optimally.

The Role of Water and Other Fluids in Digestive Health

Water is essential for our survival, not just to quench our thirst but to ensure the proper functioning of our bodily systems, including the gut. Here's how water and fluids support our digestive health:

- Water is a key component in the process of breaking down food so that our body can absorb the nutrients· Just like water is needed to dissolve sugar or salt, it helps dissolve fats and soluble fiber, making it easier for the body to process these components·

- Adequate hydration ensures that the waste products of digestion move smoothly through your gut and stay soft· This is essential for preventing constipation, a common problem that can lead to discomfort and other health issues·

- The lining of our gut, which helps absorb nutrients and prevents harmful substances from leaking into our body, contains a lot of water· Keeping hydrated helps maintain the integrity of this vital barrier, supporting overall gut health·

- Water doesn't directly feed the beneficial bacteria in our gut, but it helps create an environment where they can thrive· A well-hydrated gut allows these bacteria to move and multiply effectively, contributing to a balanced microbiome·

- Water is involved in transporting dissolved nutrients and minerals throughout our body· By staying hydrated, we ensure that the absorbed nutrients from our food reach the cells that need them, supporting our overall health·

While water is the best source of hydration, other fluids like herbal teas and broths also contribute to our daily water intake and offer additional benefits for gut health· For example, herbal teas can provide soothing relief for digestive discomfort, while bone broth contains nutrients that support gut healing and integrity·

However, it's important to be mindful of beverages that can negatively impact hydration and gut health, such as caffeinated drinks and alcohol· These can lead to dehydration and disrupt the balance of gut bacteria· Moderation is key, and focusing on water and beneficial fluids can significantly support your digestive system·

In summary, ensuring adequate hydration is a simple yet effective way to support your digestive health· By drinking enough water and incorporating beneficial fluids into your diet, you're taking a crucial step toward maintaining a healthy, well-functioning gut, which is foundational to your overall well-being·

Part IV: Practical Tips for Gut Health

Meal Planning for a Healthy Gut

Creating a meal plan focused on gut health involves selecting foods that support a diverse and thriving microbiome. This approach can help streamline your grocery shopping, reduce mealtime stress, and ensure you're consistently nourishing your body with gut-friendly foods. Here's how to get started, including some sample meal ideas and the importance of eating routines.

Sample Meal Plans and Recipes

A gut-healthy meal plan includes a variety of foods rich in fiber, probiotics, and prebiotics, along with plenty of hydration. Here are some ideas to inspire your meal planning:

Breakfast

Start with a bowl of oatmeal topped with berries and a dollop of yoghurt · The oats are a great source of prebiotic fiber, berries provide antioxidants, and the yoghurt adds a probiotic boost·

Lunch

Prepare a mixed salad with leafy greens, chopped vegetables, a handful of walnuts, and chickpeas or grilled chicken for protein· Dress it with olive oil and lemon juice· This meal is packed with fiber, healthy fats, and protein, all of which support a healthy gut·

Dinner

Try a stir-fry with a variety of vegetables like bell peppers, broccoli, and carrots, served over quinoa or brown rice· Add tofu or fish for protein· The diverse range of vegetables provides different types of fiber and nutrients, while quinoa adds additional fiber and protein·

Snacks

Opt for snacks like a sliced apple with almond butter, carrot sticks with hummus, or a small serving of mixed nuts· These provide fiber and healthy fats to keep your gut and you satisfied between meals·

Eating Routines and Gut Health

Establishing regular eating routines can significantly benefit your gut health· Eating at consistent times helps regulate your body's digestive processes, making it easier to digest and absorb nutrients effectively· Here are some tips you can include in your routine:

Eat Mindfully: Take the time to enjoy your meals without distractions· Eating slowly and chewing thoroughly can improve digestion and absorption of nutrients·

Stay Hydrated: Drink water throughout the day, aiming for at least 8 glasses· Proper hydrations is essential for digestion and keeping the gut lining healthy·

Balance Your Meals: Ensure each meal includes a good balance of fiber, protein, and healthy fats· This combination supports gut health by providing the necessary nutrients for a healthy microbiome and aiding in digestion·

Listen to Your Body: Pay attention to how different foods affect your digestion and overall well-being· Everyone's microbiome is unique, so what works for one person may not work for another·

Meal planning for a healthy gut doesn't have to be complicated· By incorporating a variety of gut-friendly foods into your diet, staying hydrated, and eating at regular intervals, you can support your digestive health and overall well-being· Remember, the goal is to create a sustainable eating pattern that includes foods you enjoy while nourishing your gut microbiome·

Lifestyle Adjustments for Optimal Gut Health

Taking care of your gut involves more than just eating the right foods· Your overall lifestyle plays a huge role in maintaining a healthy gut microbiome· Let's learn how managing stress, getting enough sleep, and staying active can contribute to optimal gut health·

Stress Management Techniques

Stress can have a big impact on your gut health· When you're stressed, your body produces stress hormones that can upset your digestive system· Here are some ways to manage stress:

- Taking slow, deep breaths can help calm your mind and reduce stress· Try to take a few minutes each day to focus on your breathing·

- Physical activity is great for reducing stress· It doesn't have to be intense; even a daily walk can help clear your mind·

- Practicing mindfulness or meditation can help you stay present and reduce stress· There are many free apps and online resources to get started·

- Engage in activities you enjoy, whether it's reading, gardening, painting, or anything else that makes you feel good·

Importance of Sleep

Good sleep is crucial for gut health· While you sleep, your body repairs itself, which includes taking care of your gut· Here's how to ensure you get enough quality sleep:

Create a Sleep Schedule: Try to go to bed and wake up at the same time every day to regulate your body's internal clock·

Reduce your Screen Time Before Bed: The blue light from screens can disrupt your sleep cycle. Try to avoid screens at least an hour before bedtime.

Create a Relaxing Bedtime Routine: Activities like reading a book, taking a warm bath, or listening to calming music can signal to your body that it's time to wind down.

Make Your Bedroom Comfortable: Ensure your sleeping environment is conducive to rest, with a comfortable mattress, minimal noise, and a cool temperature.

Physical Activity

Regular exercise is not just good for your muscles and heart, but also your gut. It helps with digestion and encourages a healthy balance of gut bacteria. Here's how to incorporate exercise into your life:

Find Activities You Enjoy: You're more likely to stick with exercise if you enjoy it. This could be anything from dancing to biking to playing a sport.

Incorporate Movement into Your Day: Take the stairs instead of the elevator, go for a walk during lunch, or do a quick workout in the morning.

Set Realistic Goals: Begin with small, achievable goals and gradually raise the intensity and duration of your workouts.

Stay Consistent: Try to be active most days of the week, even if it's just a short walk or a stretching session.

Combining a balanced diet with stress management, quality sleep, and regular physical activity creates a powerful foundation for gut health· By making these lifestyle adjustments, you can support your digestive system, promote a healthy balance of gut bacteria, and enhance your overall well-being·

Supplements and Gut Health

While a balanced diet is the best way to support gut health, sometimes our bodies might need a little extra help· This is where supplements, especially probiotics and prebiotics, can play a role· Let's learn how these supplements work and figure out when it might be a good idea to include them in your routine·

Navigating the World of Probiotic and Prebiotic Supplements

Probiotic Supplements are like reinforcements you send in to boost the number of good bacteria in your gut· These supplements contain live bacteria that are similar to the beneficial microorganisms found in your gut microbiome· Taking probiotic supplements can help replenish and diversify your gut's good bacteria, especially after it's been disturbed by factors like a course of antibiotics, poor diet, or stress·

When choosing a probiotic supplement, consider the following:

- Look for supplements with a variety of bacterial strains, as different strains have different benefits·

- Check the number of live organisms in the supplement, often listed as CFUs (colony-forming units) · A higher number doesn't always mean better, but it can indicate the supplement's potency·

- Choose supplements from reputable brands that have good reviews and are transparent about their ingredients and manufacturing processes·

Prebiotic Supplements, on the other hand, are like food for your existing good bacteria· These supplements contain fibers and other nutrients that help feed and stimulate the growth of beneficial bacteria in your gut· Prebiotics can help improve the balance of your gut microbiome, supporting overall gut health·

When selecting prebiotic supplements, look for:

- Ensure the supplement contains dietary fibers that are known to act as prebiotics, such as inulin, fructooligosaccharides (FOS), or galactooligosaccharides (GOS)·

- Choose a prebiotic that matches your dietary needs and does not cause any discomfort or allergic reactions·

When to Consider Supplements

Supplements can be helpful in certain situations, such as:

After Antibiotic Use: Antibiotics can disrupt your gut microbiome. Probiotic supplements might help restore the balance of good bacteria.

Digestive Issues: If you're experiencing persistent digestive problems, such as bloating, gas, or irregular bowel movements, probiotics and prebiotics might help regulate your digestive system.

Dietary Restrictions: If you have a restricted diet due to allergies, intolerances, or personal choices that make it difficult to get enough probiotic and prebiotic-rich foods, supplements can help fill the gap.

Immune Support: Since a significant part of the immune system is linked to the gut, maintaining a healthy microbiome with the help of supplements can support immune health.

Before starting any supplement, it's a good idea to talk with a healthcare provider, especially if you have existing health conditions or are taking other medications. They can help you choose the right supplement based on your specific needs and health goals.

Incorporating probiotic and prebiotic supplements into your routine can be a helpful way to support your gut health, but remember, they work best as part of a holistic approach that includes regular exercise, balanced diet, adequate sleep, and stress management.

Part V: Addressing Common Gut Health Issues

Identifying and Managing Food Intolerances

Food intolerances can be tricky· Unlike food allergies, which cause immediate and often severe reactions, intolerances affect your digestion and can lead to discomfort, bloating, and other gut issues· Understanding and managing food intolerances involves a careful process of elimination and reintroduction of certain foods to pinpoint what's causing the trouble·

Elimination Diets and Their Role

An elimination diet is like being a detective with your food. It's about removing certain foods from your diet that you suspect might be causing issues. The idea is to clear your system of these foods completely, to see if your symptoms improve. This process can help identify food intolerances by monitoring changes in how you feel.

Here's how to do it:

Start by Removing Common Culprits: Foods known to cause issues for many people include dairy, gluten, soy, eggs, nuts, and processed sugars. You might start by eliminating these from your diet for a few weeks.

Keep a Food Diary: Write down everything you eat and note any symptoms or changes in how

you feel· This record can help you see patterns
and identify which foods might be problematic·

Reintroducing Foods and Monitoring Symptoms

After a few weeks without the eliminated foods,
you'll start bringing them back into your diet,
one at a time· This step is crucial for pinpointing
exactly which foods cause your symptoms·

Introduce One Food at a Time: Pick one food
you eliminated and eat it several times a day for
a few days, noting any changes in symptoms· If
you don't notice any negative effects, it's likely
safe for you·

Wait a Few Days Before Trying Another Food:
This gap helps ensure that any reaction is linked
to the specific food you reintroduced·

Listen to Your Body: Pay close attention to how you feel· Symptoms of food intolerance can include digestive issues like gas, bloating, or diarrhea, but also fatigue, headaches, or skin problems·

This process can be slow but is effective in identifying foods that your body struggles with· Once you know which foods cause issues, you can adjust your diet to avoid them and hopefully alleviate your symptoms·

It's a good idea to undertake this process with the guidance of a healthcare provider or a dietitian· They can provide support and ensure your diet remains balanced and nutritious while you're eliminating and reintroducing foods·

Managing food intolerances is about learning what works for your body· By carefully identifying and eliminating problem foods, you can help support your gut health and improve your overall well-being·

Part V: Addressing Common Gut Health Issues

Strategies for Common Digestive Disorders

Digestive disorders can significantly impact your quality of life, but understanding and managing them can help you find relief and improve your well-being. Here are strategies for dealing with some common digestive disorders:

Irritable Bowel Syndrome (IBS)

IBS is a common disorder that affects the large intestine, causing symptoms like cramping, abdominal pain, bloating, gas, and changes in bowel habits (diarrhea, constipation, or both). Although IBS doesn't cause changes in bowel tissue or increased risk of colorectal cancer, its symptoms can be a significant burden·

- Keeping a food diary can help identify triggers· Many find relief by reducing high-gas foods, gluten, or FODMAPs (fermentable oligo-, di-, monosaccharides, and polyols) ·

- Since stress can exacerbate IBS symptoms, strategies like exercise, meditation, and adequate sleep can be beneficial·

- Depending on your symptoms, your doctor might recommend fiber supplements for constipation or medications to ease diarrhea and abdominal pain·

Inflammatory Bowel Disease (IBD)

IBD, including Crohn's disease and ulcerative colitis, involves chronic inflammation of the digestive tract· Symptoms can include severe diarrhea, fatigue, weight loss, and abdominal pain·

Medication: IBD usually requires medication to reduce inflammation, suppress the immune system, or treat infection· Biologics are a newer type of treatment that can be effective for some patients·

Surgery: In severe cases, surgery might be required to take out damaged parts of the digestive tract·

Diet and Nutrition: While diet doesn't cause IBD, certain foods can trigger symptoms· A low-residue or low-fiber diet may be recommended during flare-ups to reduce the frequency of bowel movements.

Other Common Digestive Issues

Many other conditions can affect digestive health, including heartburn, GERD (gastroesophageal reflux disease), and gastritis.

Lifestyle Changes: Avoiding large meals, not lying down right after eating, and staying away from trigger foods like spicy or fatty foods can help manage symptoms.

Medications: Over-the-counter antacids, H2 blockers, or proton pump inhibitors can reduce stomach acid and relieve heartburn and GERD symptoms.

<u>*Consult a Professional:*</u> Always consult with a healthcare provider for diagnosis and treatment tailored to your specific condition·

Managing digestive disorders often requires a multifaceted approach that includes dietary changes, stress management, medication, and sometimes surgery· It's crucial to work closely with healthcare professionals to develop a treatment plan that addresses your symptoms and improves your quality of life· Remember, what works for one person may not work for another, so it's important to find the right combination of strategies that work for you·

Part VI: The Future of Gut Health

The exploration of the gut microbiome is one of the most exciting areas in science today, offering new insights into human health and potential treatments for various diseases. Here's a glimpse into the latest advancements and what the future might hold for gut health and wellness.

The Latest in Gut Health Science

Recent years have seen incredible progress in our understanding of the gut microbiome. Scientists have discovered that the bacteria in our gut do much more than help digest food; they play a crucial role in our immune system, affect our mood and mental health, and may even influence our risk of developing diseases like obesity, diabetes, and heart disease.

One of the most significant innovations has been the development of advanced DNA sequencing technologies, allowing researchers to identify and study the vast array of microorganisms living in the human gut in much greater detail than ever before· This has led to a better understanding of the complex relationship between our diet, lifestyle, and gut microbiome·

Future Directions for Gut Health and Wellness

Looking ahead, the field of microbiome research holds exciting potential for personalized medicine· Here are a few particularly promising areas:

<u>Personalized Nutrition:</u> In the future, we might see diets tailored to our unique microbiome, optimizing gut health and preventing disease·

<u>Microbiome Therapies:</u> Researchers are exploring how altering the gut microbiome through faecal transplants, probiotics, and prebiotics can treat conditions ranging from Clostridium difficile infections to inflammatory bowel disease and even obesity.

<u>Early Disease Detection:</u> The composition of our gut microbiome might one day be used to predict the risk of developing certain diseases, allowing for earlier intervention.

<u>Mind and Mood:</u> The gut-brain axis is a hot topic, with ongoing research into how the microbiome influences mental health. This could lead to new treatments for depression, anxiety, and neurodegenerative diseases.

As we learn more about the gut microbiome, it's clear that it holds the key to unlocking many of our body's mysteries. The future of gut health research promises not only to revolutionize the way we think about diet and nutrition but also offer the potential for groundbreaking treatments for a wide range of diseases. The next few decades will undoubtedly bring fascinating discoveries, further emphasizing the importance of taking care of our gut microbiome for overall health and well-being.

Creating Your Personalized Gut Health Plan

Taking care of your gut is a personal journey, unique to each individual· By understanding your gut health and implementing long-term strategies, you can support your digestive system and overall well-being· Here's how to get started on creating a personalized plan for a healthy gut·

Assess Your Gut Health

The first step is to figure out the current state of your gut health· This involves paying attention to your body and noticing signs that might indicate imbalances, such as irregular bowel movements, frequent bloating, gas, or discomfort after eating certain foods·

For a few weeks, write down everything you eat and drink, along with any symptoms you experience· This can help you identify patterns or specific foods that might not agree with your gut·

If you suspect you have gut health issues, it's a good idea to talk to a doctor or a dietitian· They can offer advice, run tests if necessary, and help you understand your body's needs better·

Long-Term Strategies for Maintaining a Healthy Gut

Once you have a clearer picture of your gut health, you can start implementing strategies to support and maintain it· Here are some key components to consider:

✓ Eat a wide variety of foods, especially high-fiber fruits, vegetables, legumes, and whole grains· These provide the nutrients and prebiotics your gut bacteria need to thrive·

✓ Regularly incorporate foods like yoghurt, kefir, sauerkraut, and kimchi into your diet to boost your intake of probiotics·

✓ Drinking plenty of water is essential for a healthy digestive system· It helps digest food, absorb nutrients, and ensure smooth bowel movements·

✓ High-stress levels can negatively affect your gut· Find stress-reduction techniques that work for you, such as meditation, exercise, or hobbies that relax you·

✓ Physical activity can help keep your digestive system healthy and promote a balanced microbiome·

✓ Ensure you're getting 7-9 hours of quality sleep each night· Poor sleep can impact your gut health and immune system·

Creating a personalized gut health plan is about making consistent, mindful choices that support your digestive system's needs· It's not about perfection but finding a balance that works for your body and lifestyle· Over time, these strategies can help improve your gut health, which is a cornerstone of overall health and well-being· Remember, changes don't happen overnight, so be patient and kind to yourself as you work towards a healthier gut·

Appendix

Glossary of Terms

Bacteria: Tiny, single-celled organisms that live in various environments, including the human body, where they play critical roles in maintaining health and causing diseases·

Biologics: A type of medication derived from living organisms or containing components of living organisms· Used in the treatment of various conditions, including IBD, by targeting specific parts of the immune system·

Colon: Also known as the large intestine, it is the final part of the digestive system, where water is absorbed from food and the remaining waste material is stored as stool before being expelled·

Dietary Fiber: Plant-based nutrients that cannot be digested by the human body· They help regulate the body's use of sugars, helping to keep hunger and blood sugar in check, and are crucial for a healthy digestive system·

Digestive System: The group of organs responsible for the digestion and absorption of nutrients from food, including the stomach, intestines, liver, and others·

Faecal Transplant: A procedure where faecal matter, or stool, is collected from a tested donor, mixed with a solution, strained, and placed in a patient's gut via a colonoscopy, endoscopy, sigmoidoscopy, or enema to restore the balance of bacteria in the intestine·

Fermentation: A metabolic process that produces chemical changes in organic substrates through the action of enzymes· In food, it can preserve and produce beneficial enzymes, vitamins, and strains of probiotics·

FODMAPs: Acronym for Fermentable Oligosaccharides, Disaccharides, Monosaccharides, And Polyols, which are short-chain carbohydrates that are not properly absorbed in the small intestine and can cause digestive issues·

Gut Microbiome: The complex community of microorganisms (including bacteria, fungi, and viruses) living in the digestive tracts of humans and other animals, which is essential for digesting food, synthesizing nutrients, and protecting against pathogens·

Inflammatory Bowel Disease (IBD): A term mainly used to describe two conditions,

Crohn's disease and ulcerative colitis, which are characterized by chronic inflammation of the gastrointestinal (GI) tract·

Irritable Bowel Syndrome (IBS): A common disorder affecting the large intestine, causing symptoms like cramping, abdominal pain, bloating, gas, diarrhea or constipation, or both·

Prebiotics: Non-digestible food components that promote the growth of beneficial microorganisms in the intestines· They are found in foods like bananas, onions, garlic, and asparagus·

Probiotics: Live bacteria and yeasts that are good for your health, especially your digestive system· They are found in supplements and fermented foods like yoghurt, sauerkraut, and kimchi.

Short-Chain Fatty Acids (SCFAs): Fatty acids with fewer than 6 carbon atoms, which are produced by the gut microbiota during the fermentation of undigested carbohydrates and have various beneficial effects on the host's health.

Acknowledgements

As the journey of writing this book comes to a close, I find myself reflecting on the many people who have supported me along the way· This book is not just a collection of my thoughts and knowledge; it's a mosaic of contributions, encouragement, and wisdom from countless individuals·

First, I want to express my deepest gratitude to my family and friends (Annie, Bryan and Courtney) · Your unwavering support and belief in me provided the strength I needed to pursue this project· To my family, thank you for your endless love and for the sacrifices you've made, which allowed me the space and time to write· To my friends, your encouragement and the moments of laughter we shared were my sanctuary during this intense journey·

A special thanks go to the healthcare professionals, scientists, and researchers whose tireless work in the field of gut health has been both the foundation and inspiration for this book· Your dedication to understanding the complexities of the human body is truly awe-inspiring· I am grateful for the wealth of knowledge you have shared with the world and with me·

To the individuals who bravely shared their personal stories of struggle and triumph over digestive disorders, thank you· Your stories are a powerful reminder of why this work matters· You've shown us the strength of the human spirit, and your experiences have illuminated the pages of this book with hope and resilience·

I must also acknowledge the incredible community of dietitians, nutritionists, and health coaches whose insights into gut health and wellness have been invaluable· Your commitment to helping others achieve their healthiest selves is a beacon of light in this field·

To my editor and the publishing team, your expertise, patience, and guidance transformed my manuscript into a book I am truly proud of· Your dedication to maintaining the integrity of the work while ensuring its accessibility to all readers has been remarkable·

Finally, to you, the reader, thank you for embarking on this journey with me· This book was written for you, with the hope that it will guide you toward a healthier, happier life by understanding and nurturing your gut health· Your curiosity, willingness to learn, and commitment to your well-being are what makes all of this worthwhile·

This book is a testament to the power of community, knowledge, and shared experiences· Thank you all for being a part of this journey· Here's to our continued health and wellness·

With deepest gratitude,

DAISY HOULE

Gut Health Progress Tracker

Today's Date: _______________

Breakfast

Drinks & Snacks

Lunch

Dinner

Today I Am Feeling...

Gut Health Progress Tracker

Today's Date:

Breakfast

Lunch

Dinner

Drinks & Snacks

Today I Am Feeling...

Gut Health Progress Tracker

Today's Date: _______________________

Breakfast

Lunch

Dinner

Drinks & Snacks

Today I Am Feeling...

Gut Health Progress Tracker

Today's Date: _______________________

Breakfast

Drinks & Snacks

Lunch

Dinner

Today I Am Feeling...

Gut Health Progress Tracker

Today's Date: ___________________

Breakfast

Lunch

Dinner

Drinks & Snacks

- ☐
- ☐
- ☐
- ☐
- ☐
- ☐

Today I Am Feeling...

Gut Health Progress Tracker

Today's Date: _______________

Breakfast

Lunch

Dinner

Drinks & Snacks

Today I Am Feeling...

Gut Health Progress Tracker

Today's Date: _______________________

Breakfast

Lunch

Dinner

Drinks & Snacks

Today I Am Feeling...

GUT HEALTH PROGRESS TRACKER

Today's Date: ___________________________

Breakfast

Lunch

Dinner

Drinks & Snacks

Today I Am Feeling...

Gut Health Progress Tracker

Today's Date: _______________

Breakfast

Lunch

Dinner

Drinks & Snacks

Today I Am Feeling...

Gut Health Progress Tracker

Today's Date:

Breakfast

Lunch

Dinner

Drinks & Snacks

Today I Am Feeling...

Gut Health Progress Tracker

Today's Date: _______________________

Breakfast

Drinks & Snacks

Lunch

Dinner

Today I Am Feeling...

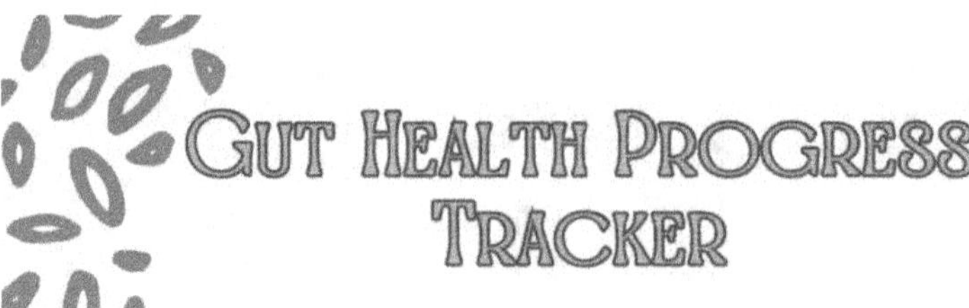

Gut Health Progress Tracker

Today's Date: _______________________________

Breakfast

Drinks & Snacks

Lunch

Dinner

Today I Am Feeling...

GUT HEALTH PROGRESS TRACKER

Today's Date: _______________________________

Breakfast

Lunch

Dinner

Drinks & Snacks

Today I Am Feeling...

GUT HEALTH PROGRESS TRACKER

Today's Date: _______________________________

Breakfast

Drinks & Snacks

- [ ] _______________________________
- [ ] _______________________________
- [ ] _______________________________
- [ ] _______________________________
- [ ] _______________________________
- [ ] _______________________________

Lunch

Dinner

Today I Am Feeling...

Gut Health Progress Tracker

Today's Date: ______________________

Breakfast

Lunch

Dinner

Drinks & Snacks

Today I Am Feeling...

GUT HEALTH PROGRESS TRACKER

Today's Date:

Breakfast

Drinks & Snacks

Lunch

Dinner

Today I Am Feeling...

GUT HEALTH PROGRESS TRACKER

Today's Date: _______________________

Breakfast

Drinks & Snacks

Lunch

Dinner

Today I Am Feeling...

Gut Health Progress Tracker

Today's Date: _______________________

Breakfast

Drinks & Snacks

Lunch

Dinner

Today I Am Feeling...

Gut Health Progress Tracker

Today's Date: _______________________

Breakfast

Drinks & Snacks

Lunch

Dinner

Today I Am Feeling...

Gut Health Progress Tracker

Today's Date: _______________________

Breakfast

Lunch

Dinner

Drinks & Snacks

Today I Am Feeling...

Gut Health Progress Tracker

Today's Date:

Breakfast

Drinks & Snacks

Lunch

Dinner

Today I Am Feeling...

Gut Health Progress Tracker

Today's Date: _______________________

Breakfast

Drinks & Snacks

Lunch

Dinner

Today I Am Feeling...

Gut Health Progress Tracker

Today's Date: __________________________________

Breakfast

Lunch

Dinner

Drinks & Snacks

- [ ] __________________________________
- [ ] __________________________________
- [ ] __________________________________
- [ ] __________________________________
- [ ] __________________________________
- [ ]

Today I Am Feeling...

GUT HEALTH PROGRESS TRACKER

Today's Date:

Breakfast

Lunch

Dinner

Drinks & Snacks

Today I Am Feeling...

Gut Health Progress Tracker

Today's Date: _______________________________

Breakfast

Drinks & Snacks

Lunch

Dinner

Today I Am Feeling...

Gut Health Progress Tracker

Today's Date: ___________________________

Breakfast

Drinks & Snacks

Lunch

Dinner

Today I Am Feeling...

Gut Health Progress Tracker

Today's Date: _______________

Breakfast

Lunch

Dinner

Drinks & Snacks

Today I Am Feeling...

Gut Health Progress Tracker

Today's Date:

Breakfast

Lunch

Dinner

Drinks & Snacks

Today I Am Feeling...

Gut Health Progress Tracker

Today's Date: ______________________________

Breakfast

Lunch

Dinner

Drinks & Snacks

Today I Am Feeling...

Gut Health Progress Tracker

Today's Date:

Breakfast

Lunch

Dinner

Drinks & Snacks

Today I Am Feeling...

Gut Health Progress Tracker

Today's Date:

Breakfast

Lunch

Dinner

Drinks & Snacks

Today I Am Feeling...

Gut Health Progress Tracker

Today's Date: ____________________

Breakfast

Lunch

Dinner

Drinks & Snacks

- [ ] ____________________
- [ ] ____________________
- [ ] ____________________
- [ ] ____________________
- [ ] ____________________
- [ ] ____________________

Today I Am Feeling...

Gut Health Progress Tracker

Today's Date: _______________________________

Breakfast

Lunch

Dinner

Drinks & Snacks

Today I Am Feeling...

Gut Health Progress Tracker

Today's Date: ___________________________

Breakfast

Lunch

Dinner

Drinks & Snacks

Today I Am Feeling...

Gut Health Progress Tracker

Today's Date: _______________________________

Breakfast

Drinks & Snacks

Lunch

Dinner

Today I Am Feeling...

Gut Health Progress Tracker

Today's Date: _______________________

Breakfast

Lunch

Dinner

Drinks & Snacks

Today I Am Feeling...

Gut Health Progress Tracker

Today's Date: _______________________________

Breakfast

Drinks & Snacks

Lunch

Dinner

Today I Am Feeling...

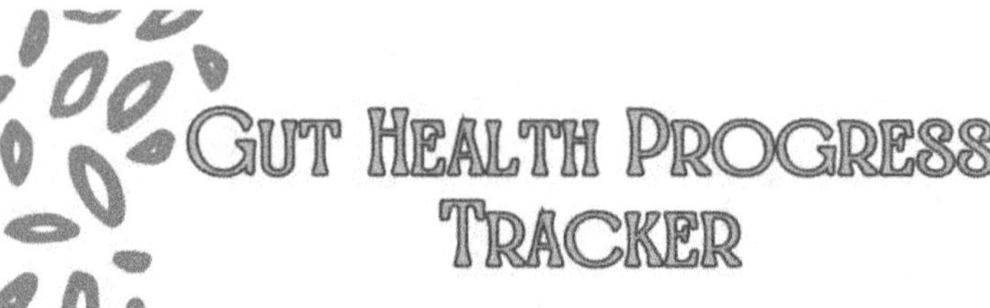

GUT HEALTH PROGRESS TRACKER

Today's Date: _______________________

Breakfast

Lunch

Dinner

Drinks & Snacks

Today I Am Feeling...

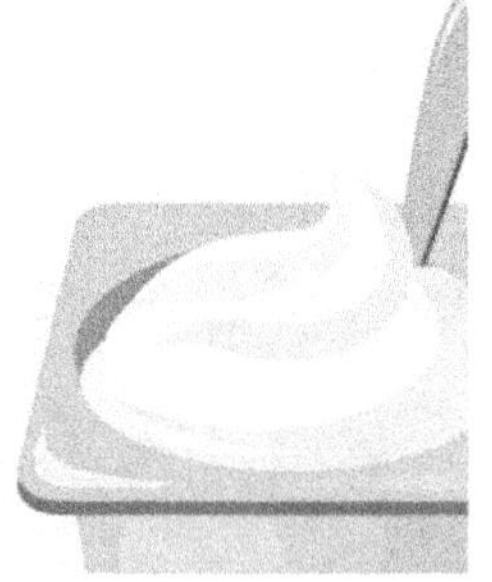

Gut Health Progress Tracker

Today's Date: ___________________________________

Breakfast

Drinks & Snacks

Lunch

Dinner

Today I Am Feeling...

Gut Health Progress Tracker

Today's Date: __________________

Breakfast

Lunch

Dinner

Drinks & Snacks

Today I Am Feeling...